Yoga Games for Kids

yoga games
for kids

**30 Fun Activities to
Encourage Mindfulness,
Build Strength,
and Create Calm**

LANI ROSEN-GALLAGHER, M.Ed., RCYT

Illustrations by Tanya Emelyanova

ROCKRIDGE
PRESS

For general information on our other products and services or to obtain technical support, please contact our Customer Care Department within the United States at (866) 744-2665, or outside the United States at (510) 253-0500.

Rockridge Press publishes its books in a variety of electronic and print formats. Some content that appears in print may not be available in electronic books, and vice versa.

Interior and Cover Designer: Stephanie Mautone
Art Producer: Samantha Ulban
Editor: Elizabeth Baird
Production Editor: Nora Milman
Production Manager: Michael Kay

Illustrations © 2021 Tanya Emelyanova.
Author Photo Courtesy of Zephyr Gallagher.

Paperback ISBN: 978-1-63807-324-6
eBook ISBN: 978-1-63807-219-5
R0

To my favorites: My hilarious and talented husband, Chris; my sweet yogi partner, Zephyr; and our cats, Puck and Purrsephone (aka yoga cat). Thank you for your never-ending support and love.

Contents

A Letter to Grown-Ups ix

1 Mindful and Present 1

Game 1: Flower Breath 3

Game 2: Butterfly Pose 4

Game 3: Flowering Lotus
Pose 7

Game 4: Child's Pose 8

Game 5: Fly or Hop? 11

Game 6: Mindful Dog 12

Game 7: Follow the
Butterfly 15

Game 8: Boat Ride 16

Game 9: Lizard on a Rock 19

Game 10: Ships at Sea 20

2 Strong and Focused 23

Game 11: Mountain Pose 25

Game 12: Warrior 1 Pose 26

Game 13: Warrior 2 Pose 29

Game 14: Tree Pose 30

Game 15: Volcano
Eruption! 33

Game 16: Who Lives in
My Tree? 34

Game 17: Sunshine Flow 37

Game 18: Peaceful
Warriors 38

Game 19: A Mini Forest 41

Game 20: Flying Warriors 42

3 Calm and Relaxed 45

Game 21: Cat/Cow Pose 47

Game 22: Seated Twist
Pose 48

Game 23: Happy Baby
Pose 51

Game 24: Lounge Chair
Pose 52

Game 25: Spring Cleaning 55

Game 26: Calm Kitties 56

Game 27: Wings in the
Garden 59

Game 28: Goodnight Flow 60

Game 29: Birthday Party 63

Game 30: Floating on a
Cloud 64

Yoga Pose Glossary 67

Where to Learn More about Yoga 71

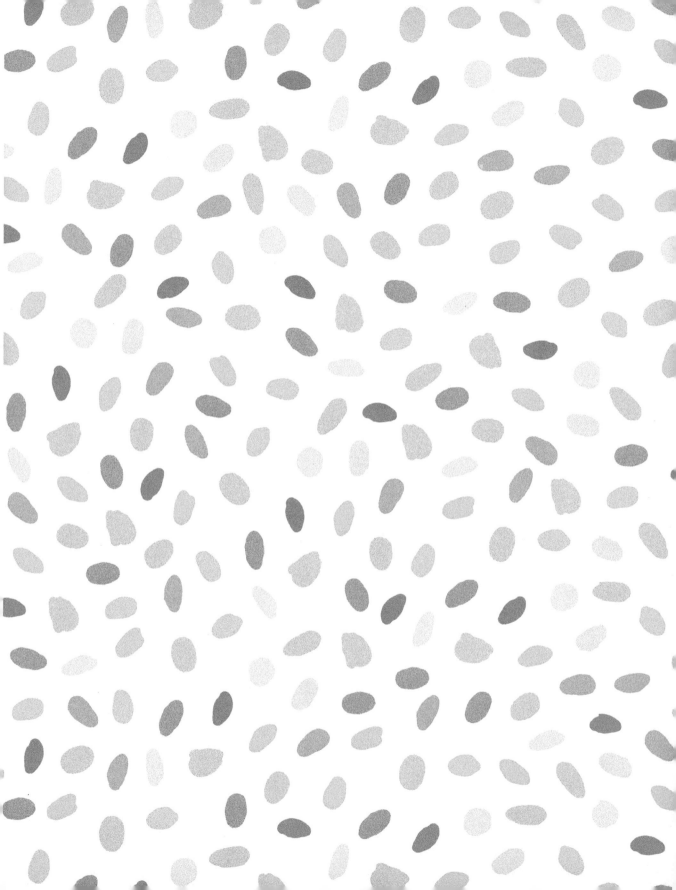

A Letter to Grown-Ups

Hi there, grown-ups!

Welcome to the joy that is practicing yoga with kids. I see yoga as an *everything* practice. It helps us balance our minds, bodies, and hearts. It's fun. It helps us find our inner strength. It is also about learning, growing, and connecting. Yoga teaches us to feel empathy for others while bringing us a sense of inner peace. It's about cultivating compassion, kindness, and trust, getting curious, and building communication. While the poses help build strength and flexibility, we also use them to take a pause, reduce stress, and find calm.

In this book, you will find 30 games that teach kids basic poses and sequences to build upon and play with. The games are meant to foster creativity and help build a routine. Coupled with each game is an affirmation that kids can say to themselves, either during the postures or anytime they want to feel a little more empowered. Each game also has a star rating to indicate how challenging or intricate it is to play. You can feel free to go in order or skip to the chapter and game that suits your child's needs that day. There is no wrong way to practice.

My favorite part of teaching is watching my students grow—when they discover how a flower breath can make them feel calm, find balance in a tough pose, or laugh in a frog hop. Each of these experiences fosters independence, resilience, and joy.

The biggest benefits will come if you can carve out a few minutes each day to practice a game or partner pose. Kids thrive on repetition; it is when a practice becomes their own. With these games, you will watch kids master new skills and build confidence. The journey doesn't stop here, but it's a great place to return to again and again. Have fun, get creative, and enjoy whatever learning unfolds!

1

Mindful and Present

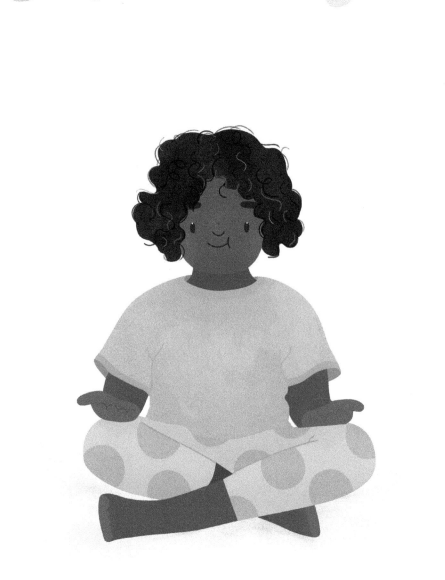

Flower Breath

Flower Breath

★☆☆

Imagine you are walking through a field of flowers. How do they smell? Sit in the middle of the field to practice calming yourself with Flower Breath.

1. Begin by sitting with your legs crossed.

2. Place your hands on your knees with your palms facing up.

3. Picture your favorite flower color.

4. Inhale and allow your fingers to come together as if flower petals were closing.

5. Exhale and allow your fingers to open as if flower petals are opening.

6. Practice this breath at least three times.

I am rooted and bright.

Butterfly Pose

⭐☆☆

Imagine you are a beautiful butterfly as you practice Butterfly Pose! You have just come out of your chrysalis with your brand-new wings. You are looking for a flower to rest on. What color are your wings?

1. Take a seat and place the bottoms of your feet together.

2. Bend your elbows and bring your hands to your shoulders.

3. Picture your beautiful butterfly wings.

4. Flap your elbows as you move your knees up and down.

5. Next, bring your hands to your feet and your nose to your toes as you hide inside your wings to rest on a flower.

6. Practice this flying and hiding at least three times.

I am patient as I grow and change.

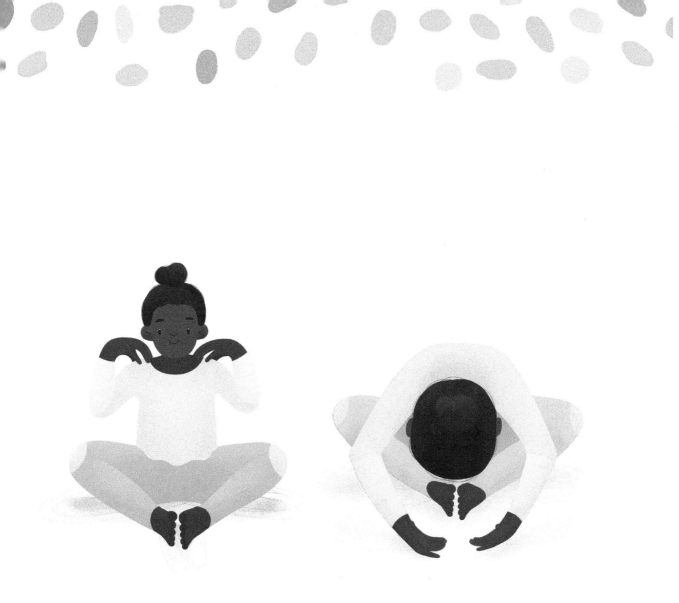

Butterfly Pose Step 1   Butterfly Pose Step 2

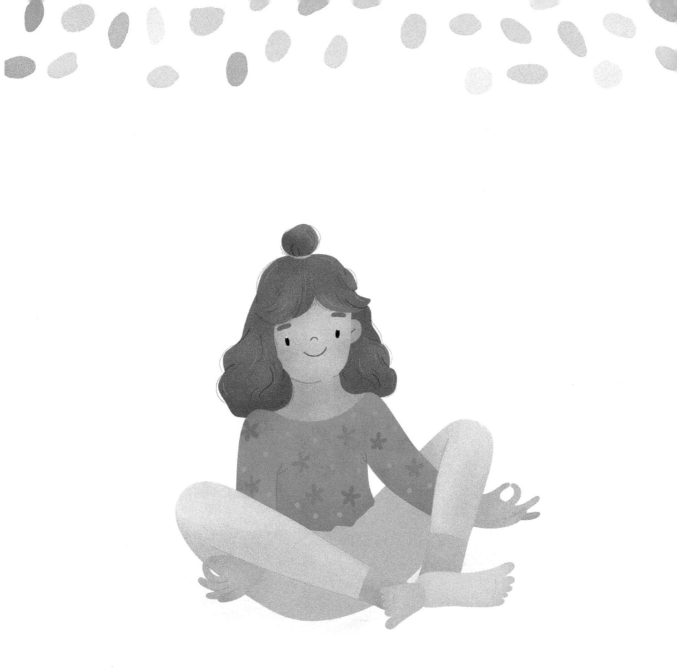

Flowering Lotus Pose

Flowering Lotus Pose

★★☆

Imagine you are a beautiful flower, a lotus (also known as a water lily). You are going to balance on the water as your petals wave in the wind while you practice Flowering Lotus Pose.

1. Begin by sitting on the ground and placing the bottoms of your feet together.

2. Bring your palms together to your heart.

3. Lift your feet and balance on your bottom.

4. Slide one palm under each of your knees as you balance.

5. Wiggle your fingers and toes as if they were the petals of a flower.

6. Picture your favorite flower color as you balance. Try to hold the pose while you inhale and exhale three times.

I like who I am, just the way I am.

Game 4

Child's Pose

⭐︎☆☆

Take a rest with Child's Pose. This is a great pose to help you find a moment of calm anytime you need a break.

1. Begin on your hands and knees.

2. Open your knees wide and touch your big toes together.

3. With a big breath, sit back on your heels.

4. Roll your upper body down toward the floor, resting your chest on the floor between your thighs.

5. Keep your arms stretched out in front of you.

6. Rest your forehead on the floor as you inhale and exhale three times.

7. Inhale and exhale again as you roll back up to sit on your heels.

I slow down and rest when needed.

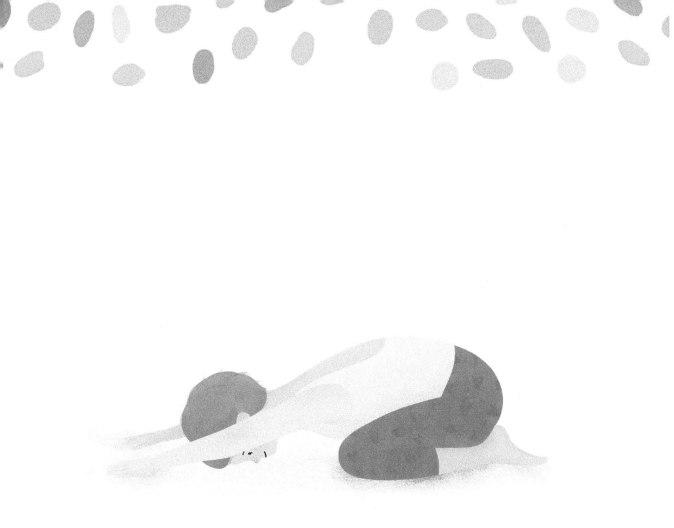

Child's Pose

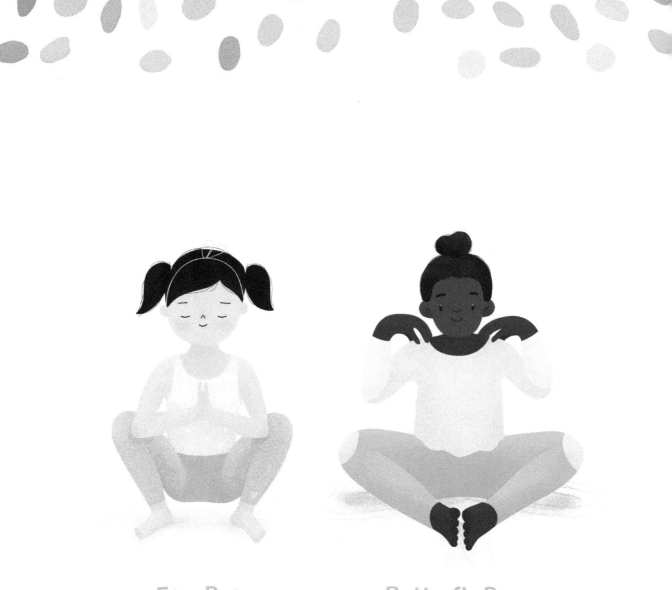

Frog Pose

Butterfly Pose

I am a part of this amazing earth.

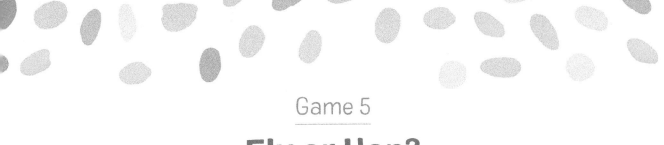

Game 5

Fly or Hop?

★★☆

What is the difference between a butterfly and a frog? One flies and the other hops! You will do two poses in this game: Butterfly Pose, from Game 2, and Frog Pose, which you'll learn here. Once you know how to do both poses, listen for the words "fly" or "hop." You will do the pose when it is called! This game can be played with a group.

Frog Pose

1. Stand with your feet as wide as your shoulders.

2. Squat down so your knees are bent and your bottom is almost to the floor.

3. Bring your palms together to your heart, like a peaceful frog.

4. Hop three times. You're a hopping frog!

5. Practice the pose a couple of times.

Play the Game

1. One person asks, "Do butterflies fly or hop?"

2. Everyone says, "Fly!" and does Butterfly Pose (Game 2).

3. The same person asks, "Do frogs fly or hop?"

4. Everyone says, "Hop!" and does Frog Pose.

5. A new person now gets to choose, and says "Fly" or "Hop." Everyone else does the pose to go with the direction!

6. Play at least five rounds.

Game 6

Mindful Dog

★★☆

Here we'll take a closer look at how you're feeling. When you practice Downward Dog Pose, you can stretch all of your body parts! As you move from one pose into the other, notice where you need extra love and give those body parts some more attention.

Downward Dog Pose

1. Begin on your hands and knees.

2. Lift your knees off the ground. Push your tail high to the sky and wag it from side to side.

3. Walk your dog by bending one knee and then the other. Let out a little "woof" if you want!

4. Inhale and exhale three times.

Play the Game

1. Begin in Child's Pose (Game 4). Take a few breaths to notice how your body feels and which body parts may need a stretch.

2. Lift your hips and come into Downward Dog Pose.

3. Walk your dog by bending one knee and then the other, and give a little "Woof!"

4. Breathe into all the parts of your body that need an extra stretch.

5. When you are ready, come back into Child's Pose (Game 4). Repeat as needed.

I listen to my body and pay attention to how I feel.

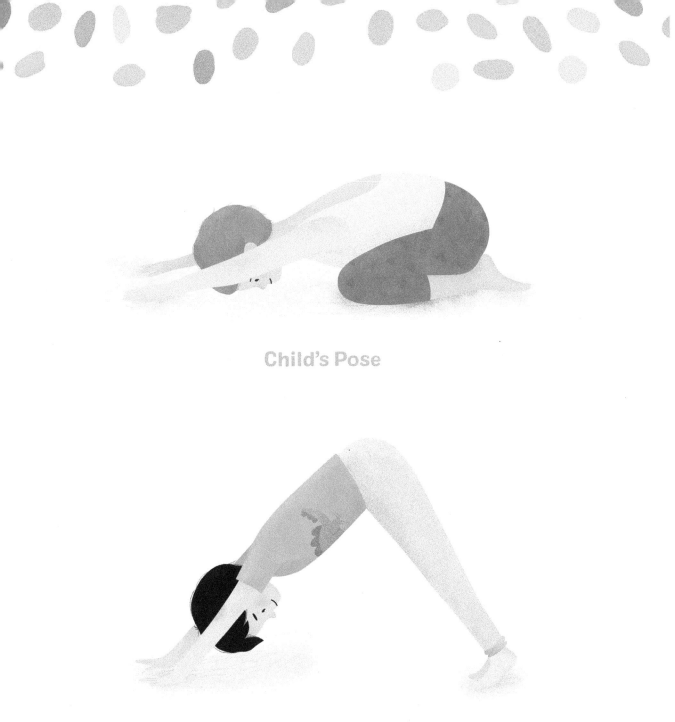

Child's Pose

Downward Dog Pose

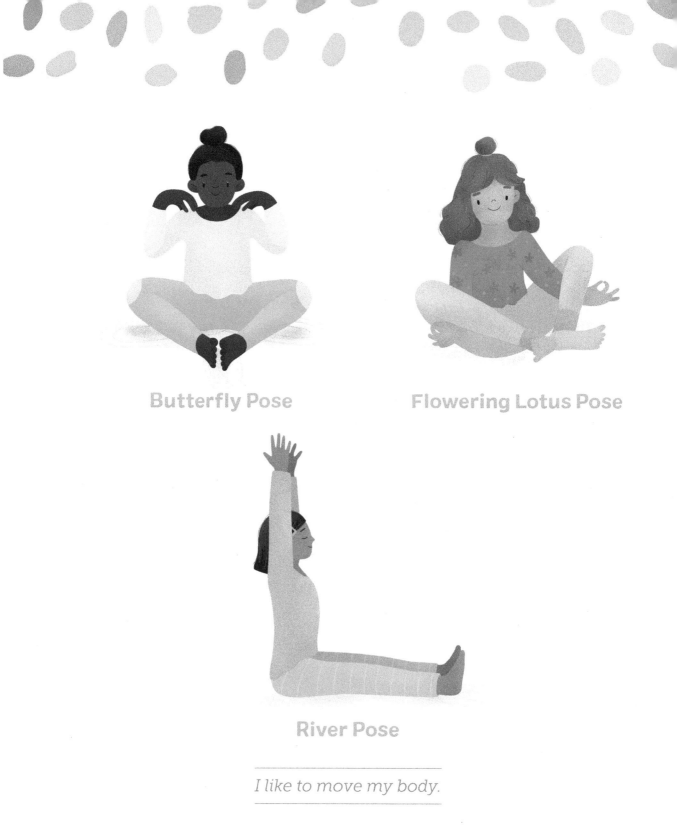

Butterfly Pose

Flowering Lotus Pose

River Pose

I like to move my body.

Follow the Butterfly

★★☆

This is a yoga version of the game Follow the Leader. To play, pick a leader from the group to start the game. Everyone will get a turn. The leader begins with one pose and everyone follows with the same pose.

River Pose

1. Begin by sitting on your bottom and stretching your legs straight out in front of you.

2. Inhale and stretch your arms up to the sky.

3. Exhale and bring your arms down to your sides like a flowing river.

4. Repeat this pose three times.

Play the Game

1. The leader does Butterfly Pose (Game 2) and says, "Butterfly."

2. Everyone follows the leader.

3. The leader does Flowering Lotus Pose (Game 3) and says, "Flower."

4. Everyone follows the leader.

5. The leader does River Pose and says, "River."

6. Everyone follows the leader.

7. The leader mixes up the order for two more rounds.

8. Now a new leader takes over. The game continues until everyone's been a leader. You can add any other poses you learn from the rest of the book.

Game 8

Boat Ride

★★☆

You are taking a boat ride on a river! What creature will you see on your boat ride? Get ready for your journey.

Boat Pose

1. Begin by sitting on your bottom and giving your knees a hug.
2. Point your arms straight forward as you lift each leg off the floor in front of you and balance on your bottom.
3. Your legs can be straight or bent.
4. Inhale and exhale three times as you hold this pose, releasing your feet down if needed.

Play the Game

1. Begin by sitting on your bottom.
2. Get into Boat Pose.
3. Paddle your boat down the river, sitting up tall and straight in River Pose (Game 7).
4. Do you see any creatures sitting on the banks of the river?
5. Look, there's a frog! Squat down into Frog Pose (Game 5).
6. Get back into Boat Pose and paddle home.

I am calm and balanced.

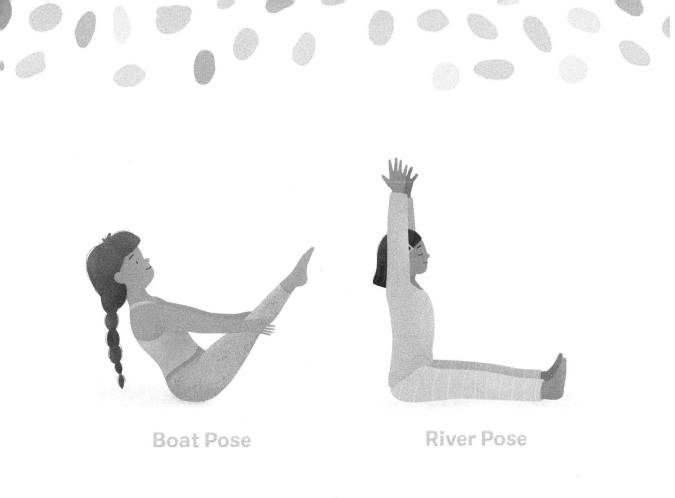

Boat Pose

River Pose

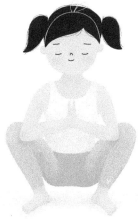

Frog Pose

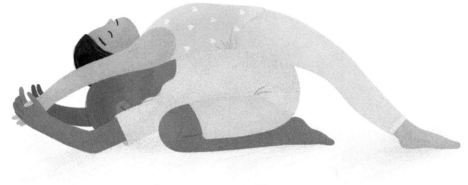

Lizard on a Rock

Lizard on a Rock

★★★

You'll want to get a partner for this game. Imagine you are at the edge of a river and you see a lizard lounging on a rock—that's you! The sun feels hot on your lizard belly as you stretch out. The larger person will be the rock and the smaller person will be the lizard. If you and your partner are similar sizes, you can take turns being the lizard. Begin Lizard on a Rock by sitting facing away from your partner.

1. The rock will come into Child's Pose (Game 4).

2. The lizard will squat at the bottom of the rock and roll their lizard back onto the rock.

3. The lizard will stretch their body along the rock as they bask in the sun!

4. "How are you, rock?" asks the lizard, reaching their hands over their head toward the floor.

5. "How are you, lizard?" asks the rock, reaching up and gently holding the lizard's hands.

6. Take a big breath in together. When you exhale, the rock and lizard will rise up together.

I take care of myself and others.

Ships at Sea

★★☆

You will want to find a partner for this game. Together, you can find balance and float on the waves in Partner Boat Pose. Begin by sitting facing your partner.

Play the Game

1. Bring your knees in to your chest with your heels as close to your body as you can.

2. Reach for your partner's hands.

3. Touch the bottoms of your feet to the bottoms of your partner's feet.

4. Now balance in this position.

5. Straighten your legs up as if you were in Boat Pose (Game 8) with your arms on the outside of your legs. You are now in Partner Boat Pose. Try to bring your legs to the outside of your arms without falling over!

6. Inhale and exhale three times as you float above the waves. Have fun by moving your arms over and under your legs as you sail along the water.

7. Bring your legs down and give your knees a hug and a squeeze.

I learn and connect with others.

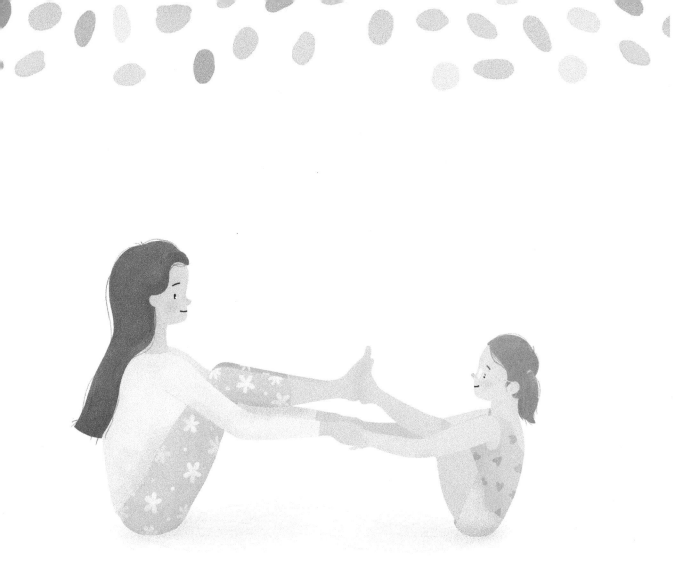

Partner Boat Pose

2
Strong and Focused

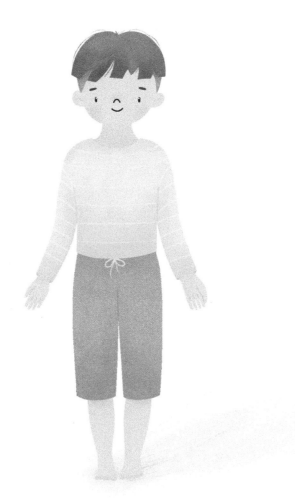

Mountain Pose

Mountain Pose

★☆☆

Imagine you are a tall and steady mountain with your feet planted into the earth as you practice Mountain Pose.

1. Stand with your feet together or hip-width apart.

2. Bring your arms down to your sides, palms open and wide, reaching your fingers to the earth.

3. As you inhale, feel your feet ground down into the earth.

4. With an exhale, roll your shoulders back and feel your spine get long.

5. Inhale and exhale three times while standing tall and steady.

I am steady like a mountain.

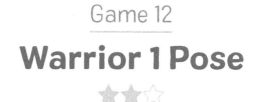

Warrior 1 Pose

★★☆

You can do anything you set your mind to! As you stand in Warrior 1 Pose, think about something that makes you feel brave.

1. Begin in Mountain Pose (Game 11).

2. Step one foot forward and the other foot back at an angle.

3. As you inhale, reach both arms up to the sky.

4. As you exhale, bend your front knee forward and stretch into your back foot.

5. Inhale and exhale two times, then say out loud, "I am brave!"

I can do anything.

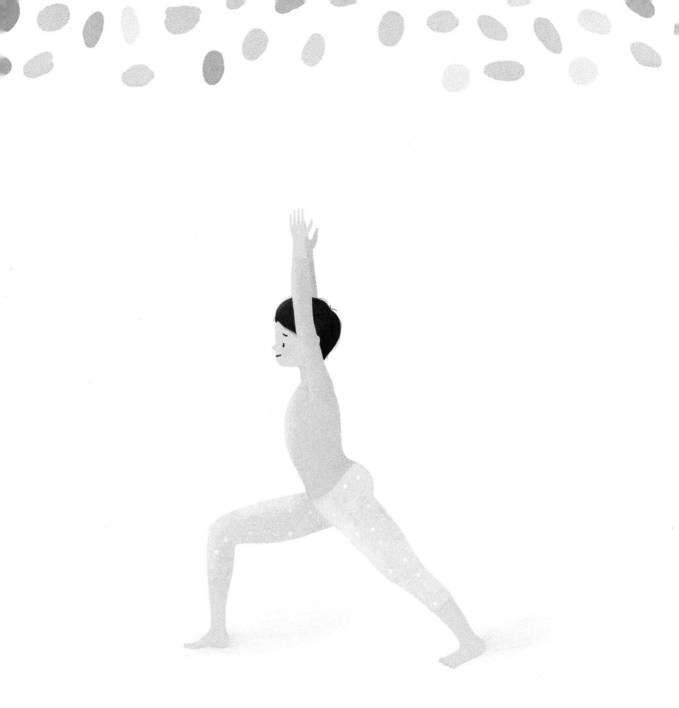

Warrior 1 Pose

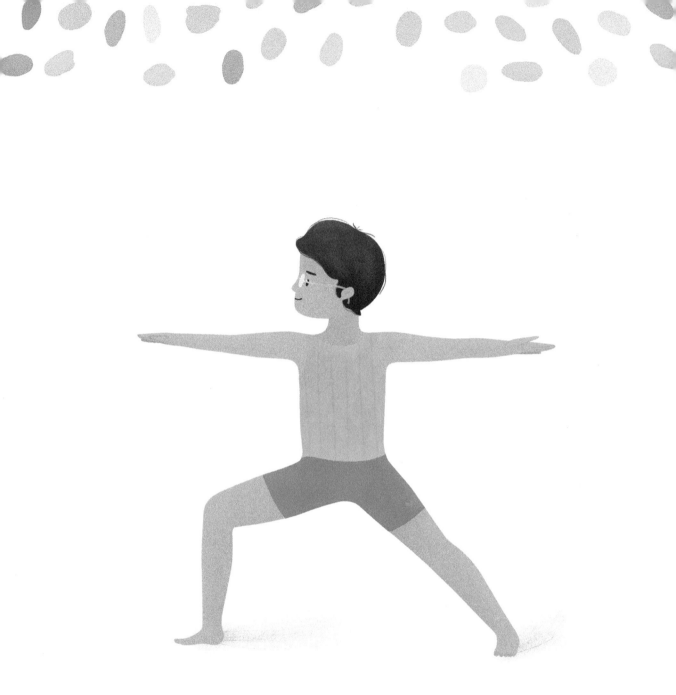

Warrior 2 Pose

Warrior 2 Pose

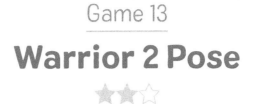

You have inner strength. As you stand in Warrior 2 Pose, think about something that makes you feel strong.

1. Begin in Warrior 1 Pose (Game 12).

2. As you inhale, stretch your arms tall to the sky.

3. As you exhale, open your arms out to either side of your body.

4. Look over your front fingers while stretching your other arm back toward your back foot.

5. Inhale and exhale two times, then say out loud, "I am strong!"

I can take on tough challenges.

Tree Pose

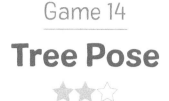

Imagine you are a strong, beautiful tree. Your roots ground you into the earth. Your branches reach toward the sky. As you balance in Tree Pose, imagine all the creatures that could live in your tree.

1. Begin in Mountain Pose (Game 11).

2. Imagine you have roots growing out of one foot, grounding you to the earth.

3. Find something to look at that is still.

4. As you inhale, bring your palms together at your heart.

5. As you exhale, begin to lift one foot and place it on your other standing leg.

6. As you inhale, lift your arms to the sky as if they were beautiful tree branches.

7. As you exhale, feel your body both lifting to the sky and grounding to the earth.

I am connected to all living things.

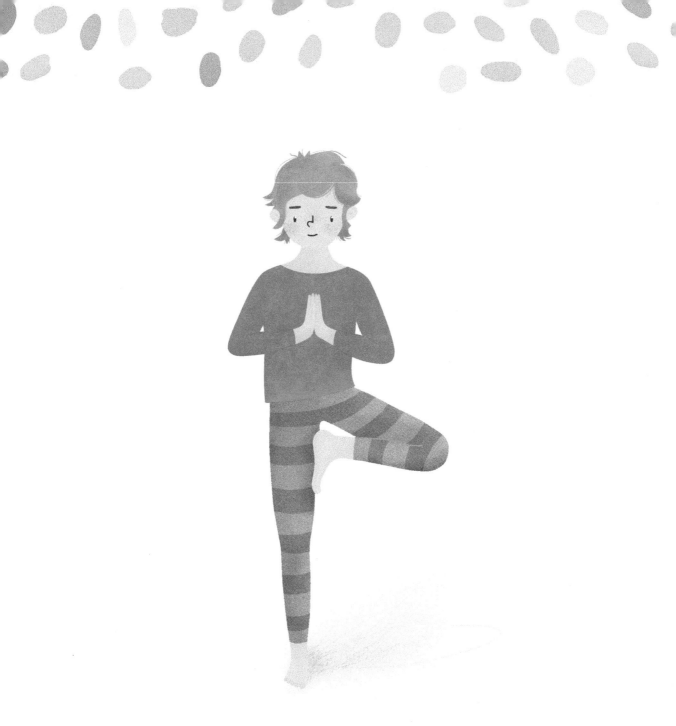

Tree Pose

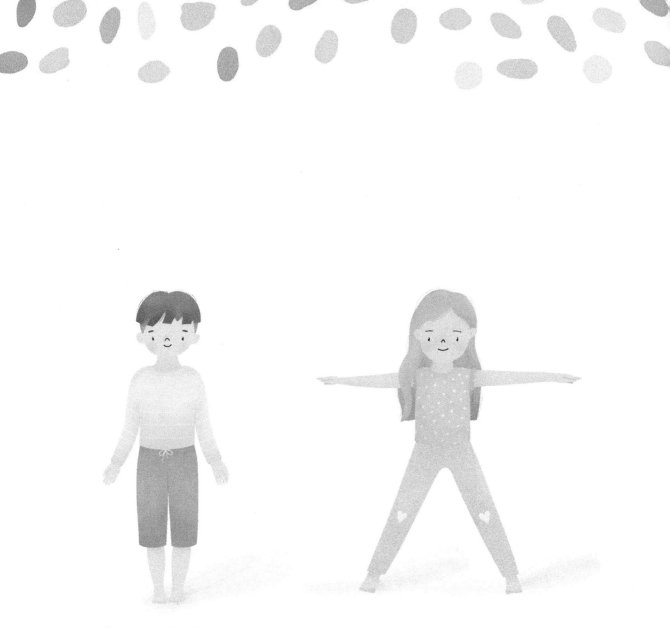

Mountain Pose

Standing Star Pose

Volcano Eruption!

★★☆

Imagine you are a tall, strong volcano as you practice Standing Star Pose. You have hot lava churning deep within. From the stillness of your mountain comes the explosion of the hot lava!

Standing Star Pose

1. Begin in Mountain Pose (Game 11).

2. Step your feet out wide beyond your shoulders.

3. Inhale and reach your arms straight out to the side.

4. Exhale and imagine your bright light shining out into the world.

5. Breathe your beautiful light in and out three times.

Play the Game

1. Begin in Mountain Pose (Game 11).

2. Bring your arms up to the sky and say, "Mountain!"

3. Bring your palms together and rub them and say, "Volllllcano!"

4. Jump your legs and arms apart and come into Standing Star Pose.

5. Jump your arms and legs back together into Mountain Pose (Game 11) and say, "Mountain!"

6. Continue to do the mountain and volcano combination two more times.

I am overflowing with love.

Who Lives in My Tree?

★ ★ ★

Imagine you are a tree, full of life. There are creatures who use your tree for their home. Can you think about which animals might live there? You can practice your flying creature poses in this game. This game can be played alone or with others.

Eagle Pose

1. Begin in Mountain Pose (Game 11).

2. Cross one leg over the other.

3. Inhale and stretch your wings out wide.

4. Exhale and cross one elbow over the other elbow and either bring your palms together or give yourself a hug.

5. Inhale and bend your knees. Lift your foot if that feels good to you!

6. Exhale and lift your elbows up to feel the stretch in your shoulders.

7. Count to three and with a big breath, open your eagle wings to stand back in Mountain Pose (Game 11).

8. Switch sides by crossing your leg the other way to start and repeat steps 3 to 7.

Play the Game

1. Begin in Tree Pose (Game 14).

2. Imagine the creatures who might use your tree for their home.

3. There is a huge nest on your branch. What flying creature could it be? Everyone goes into Eagle Pose!

4. Now what's that on your branch? Is that an owl? Squat down in Frog Pose (Game 5) and clasp your arms behind your back with your elbows out like wings.

5. Open your wide owl eyes and look around and say, "Whoooo, whoooo!"

6. Who may come to land on your tree branch next? Keep the game going by adding more poses you have learned.

I am smart and wise.

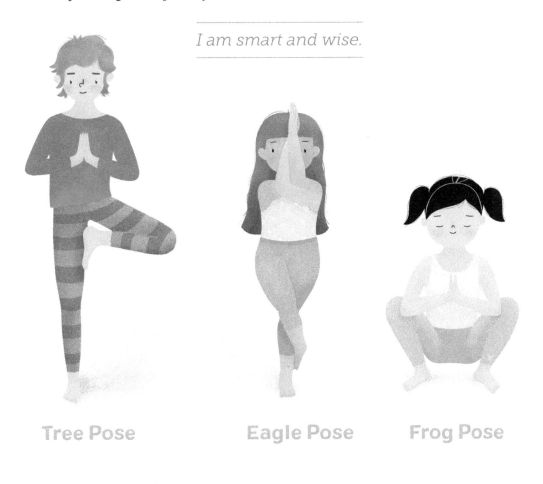

Tree Pose   Eagle Pose   Frog Pose

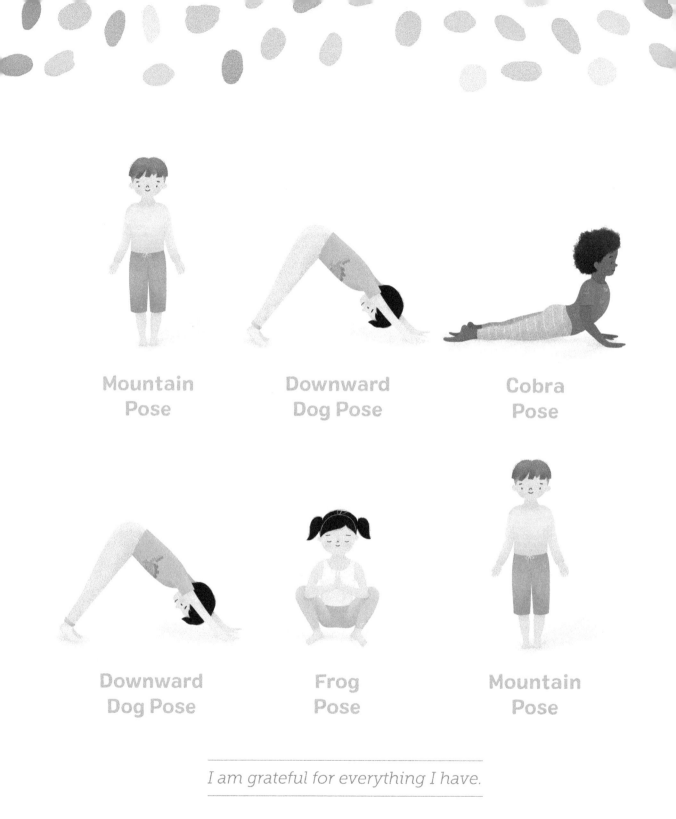

Mountain
Pose

Downward
Dog Pose

Cobra
Pose

Downward
Dog Pose

Frog
Pose

Mountain
Pose

I am grateful for everything I have.

Sunshine Flow

★ ★ ★

This is a great routine to get your day started. It's a mini sun salutation, a common yoga flow that wakes up your body and shows gratitude to the sun. It includes Cobra Pose. This game can be played alone or with others.

Cobra Pose

1. Begin on your belly with your hands placed flat on the floor under your shoulders.

2. Press into your hands to straighten your arms, keeping your shoulders down away from your ears for Cobra Pose.

3. Inhale, then with an exhale, bend your elbows, lower your body, and say, "Hisssssssss."

4. Repeat steps 1 to 3 two more times.

Play the Game

1. Begin in Mountain Pose (Game 11).

2. With an inhale, stretch your arms up to the sun and say, "Thank you, sun!"

3. As you exhale, fold your body forward and walk your feet backward into Downward Dog Pose (Game 6). Make sure to wag your tail!

4. Lower onto your belly and come into Cobra Pose.

5. Inhale and then push yourself back up into Downward Dog Pose (Game 6).

6. Exhale and then jump your feet up to your hands, getting into Frog Pose (Game 5).

7. Take one more big breath as you stretch back up into Mountain Pose (Game 11).

Peaceful Warriors

★★☆

As peaceful warriors, we are brave, strong, and kind. In this game, you will move through the warrior poses, using your breath to guide you. This game can be played alone or with others.

Peaceful Warrior Pose

1. Begin in Mountain Pose (Game 11).

2. Move into Warrior 2 Pose (Game 13).

3. Inhale and reach your back hand to your back leg and your front arm up to the sky.

4. Inhale and exhale two times, then say out loud, "I am peaceful!"

5. Take another full breath and then return to Mountain Pose (Game 11).

Play the Game

1. Begin in Mountain Pose (Game 11).

2. Inhale and move into Warrior 1 Pose (Game 12). After you exhale, say "I am brave!"

3. Inhale and move into Warrior 2 Pose (Game 13). After you exhale, say "I am strong!"

4. Inhale and reach back into Peaceful Warrior Pose. After you exhale, say "I am kind!"

5. Move your body back into Mountain Pose (Game 11) and inhale and exhale once.

6. Repeat steps 2 to 5, stepping forward with your other foot.

I am strong inside and out.

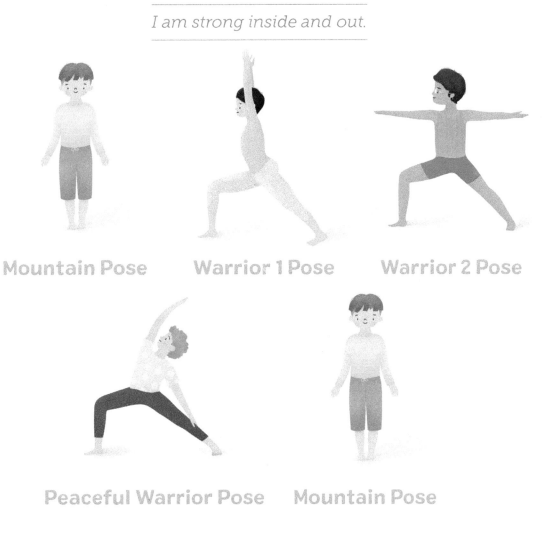

Mountain Pose   Warrior 1 Pose   Warrior 2 Pose

Peaceful Warrior Pose   Mountain Pose

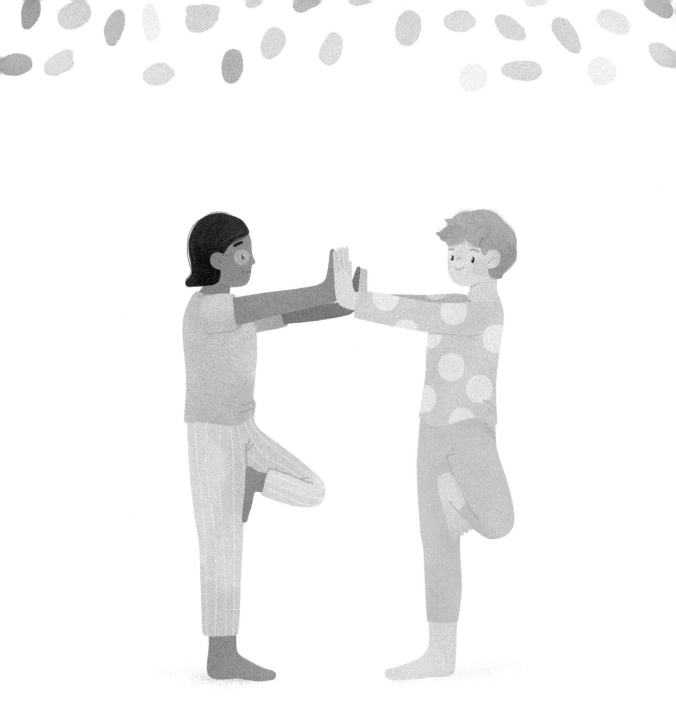

Partner Tree Pose

A Mini Forest

★★☆

Partner Tree Pose is where two people work together to form a mini forest of trees. You will help each other balance by placing your palms against your partner's palms.

Play the Game

1. Begin by facing your partner in Mountain Pose (Game 11).

2. Imagine you are rooted in the earth as you inhale. Bring your palms together to your heart for balance.

3. As you exhale, look at your partner with a big smile.

4. Bring your palms to touch your partner's palms in front of you.

5. Lift a foot off the ground and place it onto your other leg. You are now in Partner Tree Pose.

6. Continue to breathe and balance with your partner.

7. Return your foot to the ground, then repeat steps 5 and 6 with your other foot.

I like to help others.

Flying Warriors

★★☆

Imagine you are able to fly. Now you have a partner to help you! Together you will help each other balance and fly in Flying Warriors Pose.

Play the Game

1. Begin by standing next to your partner in Mountain Pose (Game 11).

2. Inhale and bring your palms together to your heart.

3. Exhale and open your arms out to your sides as if they were wings.

4. Reach for your partner's arm, back, or shoulder, and hold on!

5. Begin to lean forward together as your outer leg reaches out straight behind you.

6. When your body is parallel to the floor, find a spot to look at to keep your balance. You are now in Flying Warriors Pose.

7. Inhale and exhale three times as you imagine flying over the earth together.

8. Switch places with your partner, and repeat so that you balance on your other leg.

I am a good friend.

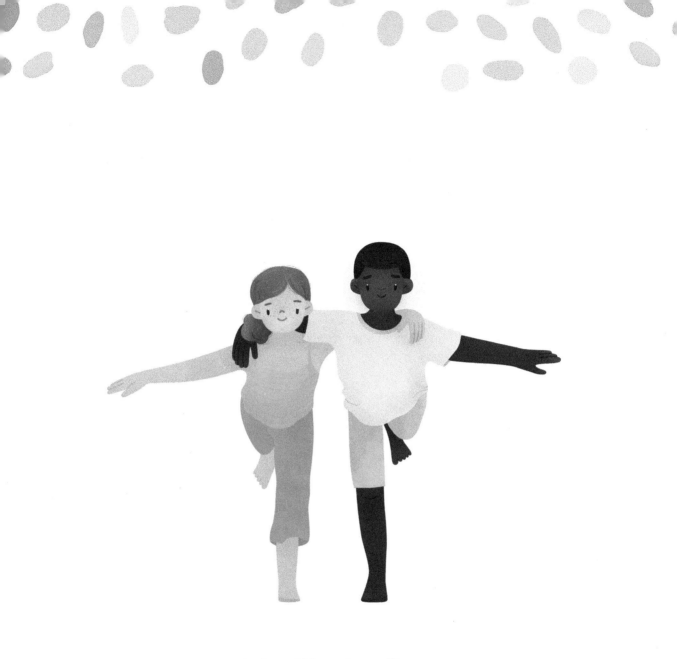

Flying Warriors Pose

3
Calm and Relaxed

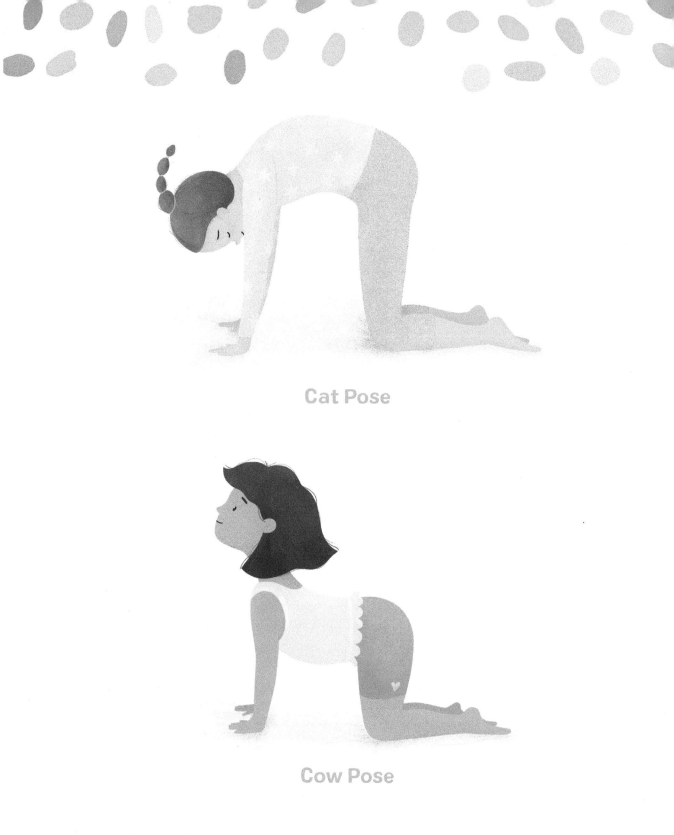

Cat Pose

Cow Pose

Cat/Cow Pose

★☆☆

Did you know that the cat and cow are best friends in yoga? They often go together as you link each pose to the other with your breath.

1. Begin on your hands and knees.

2. With an inhale, round your back up to the sky like a cat.

3. Look at your belly and let out a little "Meow." You're in Cat Pose.

4. Exhale and drop your belly toward the floor like a cow.

5. Look up to the sky and say, "Mooooo." You're in Cow Pose.

6. Continue to inhale as you round into cat pose and exhale as you drop into cow pose.

I am creative and playful.

Game 22

Seated Twist Pose

★☆☆

Imagine you could clean your body from the inside out. Seated Twist Pose will help you wring out your back like a washcloth and get rid of what you don't need. So, take a twist and let it all go!

1. Begin by sitting with your legs crossed.

2. Bring one hand to your opposite knee.

3. Bring your other hand behind your back.

4. Inhale and stretch your spine tall like a tree.

5. Exhale and look over your shoulder as you continue to twist.

6. Switch your arms to twist in the other direction, and do the Seated Twist Pose as many times as you like.

I can handle twists and turns.

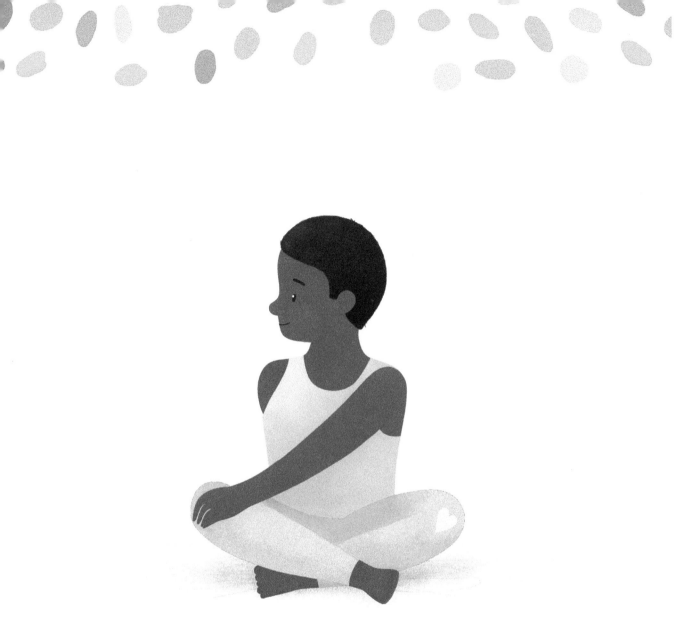

Seated Twist Pose

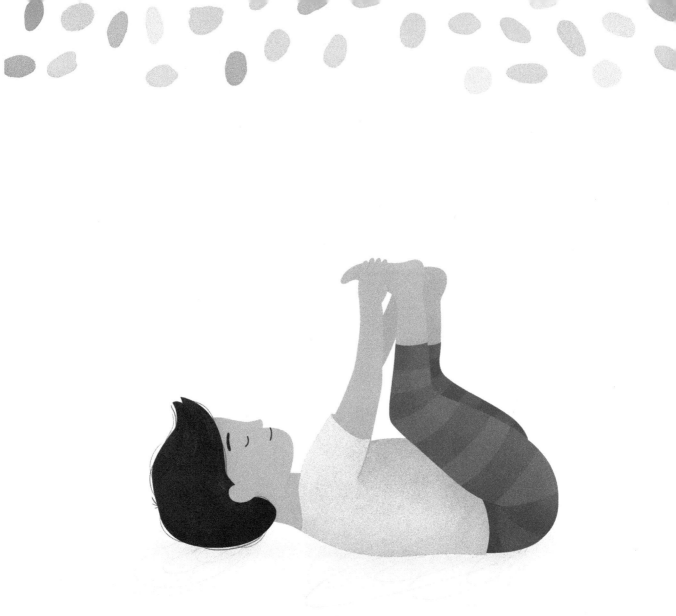

Happy Baby Pose

Happy Baby Pose

⭐☆☆

Have you ever seen how happy a baby looks when they're just laughing and playing on their back? Pretend to be a baby again as you stretch and shake out your body in Happy Baby Pose.

1. Begin by lying on your back.

2. Lift your legs and hold on to your feet.

3. While holding your feet, inhale, bending your knees and stretching your hips.

4. Exhale as you let go of your feet. Shake it all out.

5. Inhale and hold on to your feet again. Rock side to side.

6. Exhale as you let go of your feet and shake it all out one final time.

I am happy and free.

Lounge Chair Pose

★★☆

Imagine you are outside on a beautiful day sitting in a lounge chair. Find a partner who will be your chair! You and your partner will help each other practice a forward bend and a heart-opening backbend as you take turns relaxing in Lounge Chair Pose.

1. Sit back-to-back with your partner. Your legs can be straight out in front of you or crossed.

2. One partner bends forward, reaching toward their toes.

3. The other partner leans into their partner's back, bringing their arms out to the sides. Now you are lounging!

4. While lounging, imagine your heart is opening. Send love to yourself and your family from your open heart.

5. Inhale and exhale with your partner.

6. Switch so each partner gets a turn to lounge.

I am generous and openhearted.

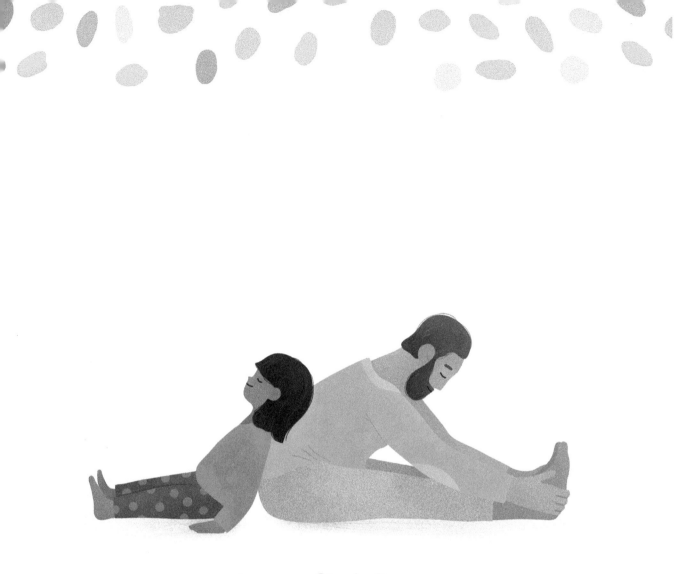

Lounge Chair Pose

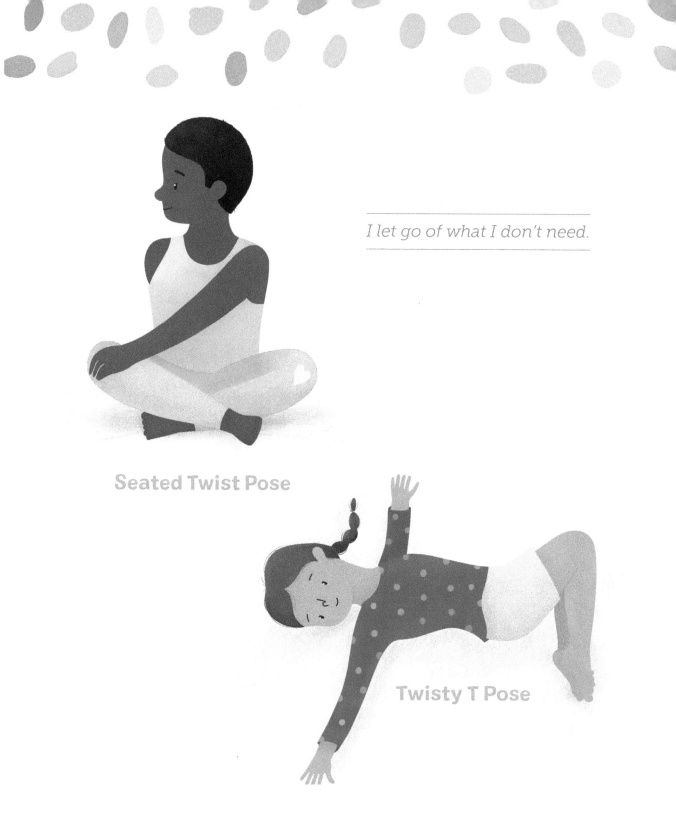

I let go of what I don't need.

Seated Twist Pose

Twisty T Pose

Spring Cleaning

★☆☆☆

Have you ever noticed that when the weather starts to get nice, the windows get opened, things get dusted, and the house gets freshly cleaned? You can also clean your body, letting go of things you don't need. When we twist in Twisty T Pose, it's like wringing water out of a washcloth.

Twisty T Pose

1. Begin by lying on your back with your legs straight out in front of you.

2. Bring your knees in to your chest with a hug and a squeeze.

3. Roll your knees over to one side.

4. Open your arms out like the letter "T."

5. Turn your head to face away from where your knees are pointing.

6. Stay here while you inhale and exhale three times.

7. Switch sides by rolling your knees over your chest to the other side and looking in the opposite direction. Breathe three more times.

Play the Game

1. Begin by sitting with your legs crossed.

2. Come into Seated Twist Pose (Game 22). Imagine you are wringing out what you do not need!

3. Roll onto your back.

4. Come into Twisty T Pose. Imagine how happy you are making all your body parts with this twist!

Calm Kitties

★☆☆

Kitties are experts at stretching and resting. Find your inner kitty as you move from Cat Pose into Cow Pose (Game 21) and then into quiet and still Child's Pose (Game 4). Use your breath to guide you as you stretch and rest like a kitty cat.

Play the Game

1. Begin on your hands and knees and move your body from Cat Pose to Cow Pose (Game 21) as you give your spine a stretch.

2. Come down into Child's Pose (Game 4). Roll your forehead side to side as you begin to quiet your mind.

3. Repeat steps 1 and 2 three more times.

I am a good listener.

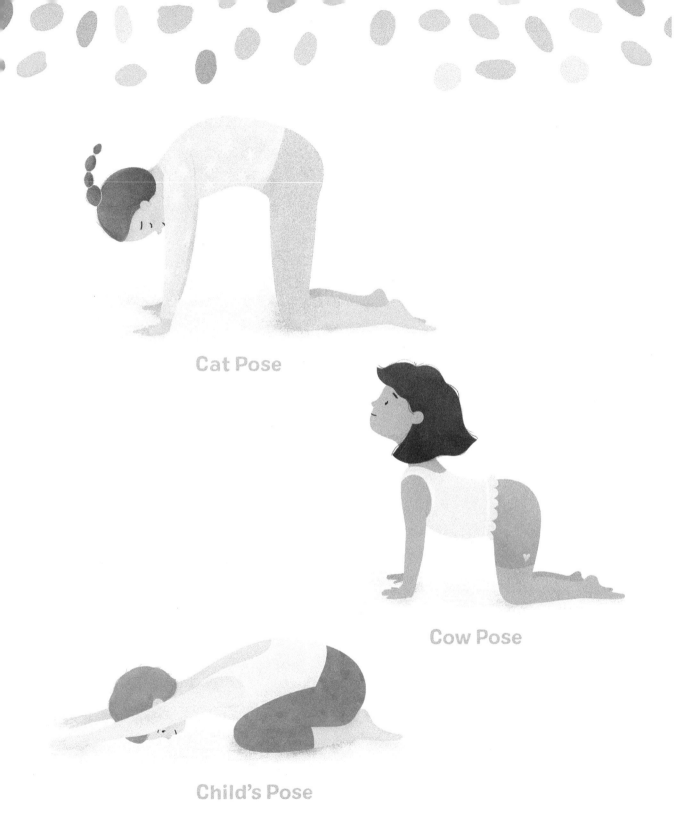

Cat Pose

Cow Pose

Child's Pose

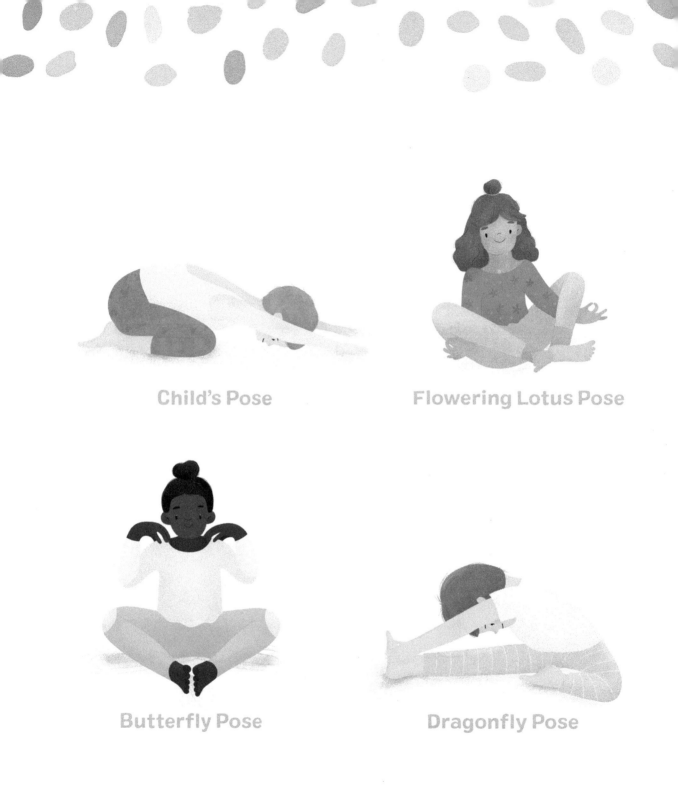

Child's Pose

Flowering Lotus Pose

Butterfly Pose

Dragonfly Pose

Wings in the Garden

★★☆

Turn your body into a little garden. Imagine turning into a seed that then grows into a beautiful flower. What creatures could you attract with your flower?

Dragonfly Pose

1. Begin sitting in River Pose (Game 7).

2. Bend one knee and bring your foot to press against the opposite thigh.

3. Inhale and stretch your arms to the sky.

4. As you exhale, fold forward and reach for your toes.

5. Repeat with the other knee.

Play the Game

1. Begin on your knees and place your head down in Child's Pose (Game 4). What kind of flower seed are you?

2. Imagine you have soil covering you. Add a little sprinkle of rain to help you grow. What else do seeds need? The sun! Feel the warmth of the sun on your back.

3. Gently roll up to sit on your bottom, then move into Flowering Lotus Pose (Game 3). Think about what kind of flower you have grown into.

4. Bring your feet down and your hands up to your shoulders as you fly into Butterfly Pose (Game 2), drinking nectar from your flower.

5. Here comes a dragonfly! Move your body into Dragonfly Pose.

I have everything I need to grow.

Goodnight Flow

★★★

End your day with this relaxing routine to calm your body. After you learn Birthday Candle Pose, you're ready to begin. Imagine your favorite flower and follow the poses to stretch your body beneath the night sky to prepare for a restful night's sleep.

Birthday Candle Pose

1. Begin on your back with your legs straight out in front of you.

2. Lift your legs up to the sky.

3. Wiggle your toes as you light your birthday candle.

Play the Game

1. Begin seated with your legs crossed.

2. Practice Flower Breath (Game 1).

3. Roll your body onto your back and lift your legs up to the sky for Birthday Candle Pose.

4. Count backward from 10 as you lower your legs and blow out your candle.

5. Hold on to your feet for Happy Baby Pose (Game 23).

6. Fold your knees over to each side to practice Twisty T Pose (Game 25).

I like to rest my brain and body after a long day.

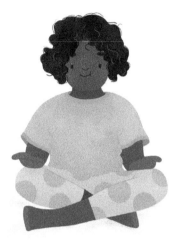

Flower Breath

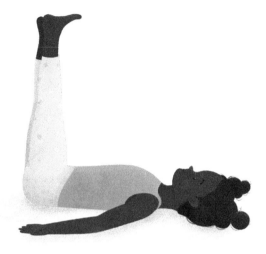

Birthday Candle Pose

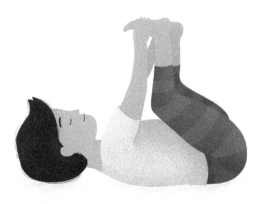

Happy Baby Pose

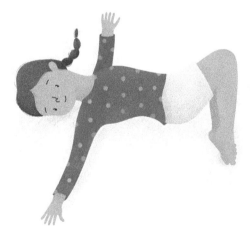

Twisty T Pose

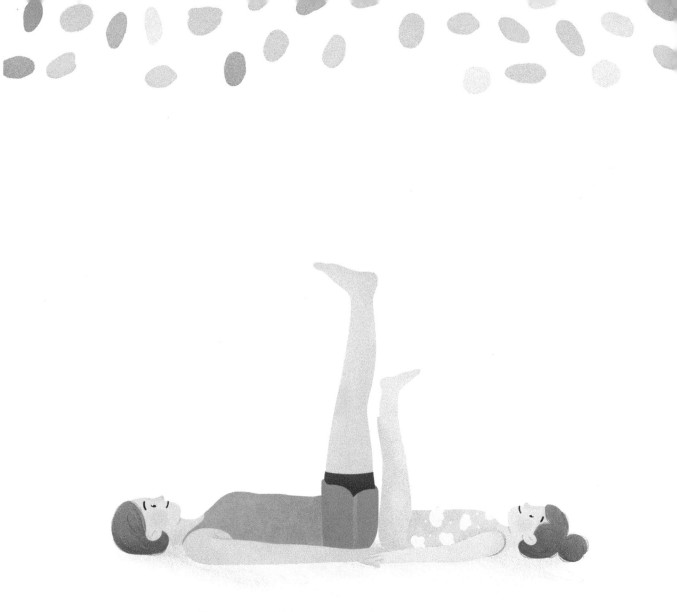

Partner Birthday Candle Pose

Birthday Party

★★☆

Pretend it's your birthday today and light a candle with a partner. You and your partner will support each other with your legs. Light your candle with your toes and then blow out your candle. Make the wish for yourself or send it to someone else!

Play the Game

1. Begin by lying on your back.

2. Both partners lift their legs to the sky into Birthday Candle Pose (Game 28).

3. Scoot your bottom against your partner's bottom as you rest your legs against each other.

4. Reach and hold your partner's hands for Partner Birthday Candle Pose. Relax as you inhale and exhale three times.

5. Now bend your knees in to your chest and bring the bottoms of your feet against your partner's feet.

6. Gently roll to the side together and then up to sit with your legs crossed.

I shine my bright light into the world.

Floating on a Cloud

⭐☆☆

Take a break on a fluffy cloud as you imagine yourself floating in Relaxation Pose. Pay attention to your breaths and find your way to calm.

Play the Game

1. Begin by lying on your back with your legs in front of you.

2. Notice how the floor feels beneath your body, and imagine you are lying on a cloud.

3. Picture this cloud, soft and fluffy, around your body.

4. Take a deep breath, then come into stillness.

5. Relax your body from the top of your head to the bottoms of your feet.

6. What sounds do you hear while you float on this cloud?

7. Take another deep breath in this Relaxation Pose.

8. When you are ready, quietly and gently roll up to sit with your legs crossed.

9. Notice how you are feeling.

I can make a difference.

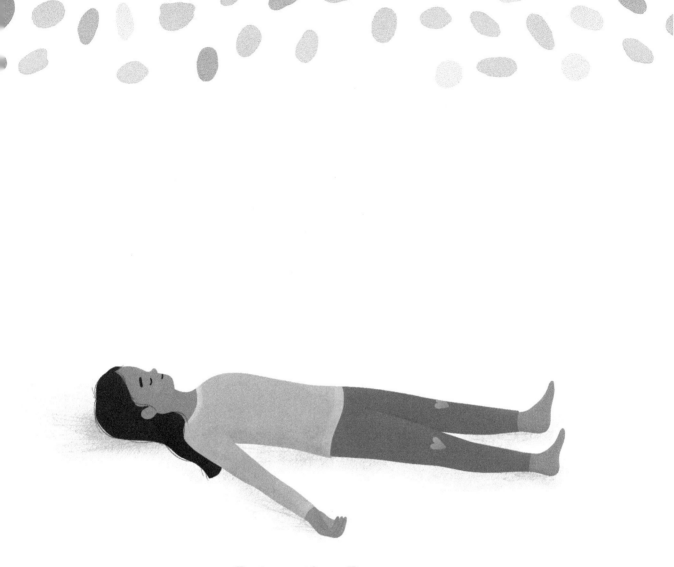

Relaxation Pose

Yoga Pose Glossary

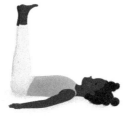

Birthday Candle Pose: *Sarvangasana*

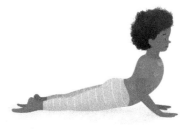

Boat Pose: *Navasana*

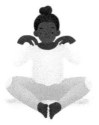

Butterfly Pose: *Baddha Konasana*

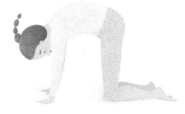

Cat Pose: *Marjaryasana*

Child's Pose: *Balasana*

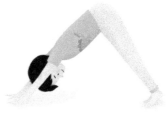

Cobra Pose: *Bhujangasana*

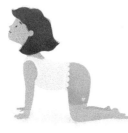

Cow Pose: *Bitilasana*

Downward Dog Pose:
Adho Mukha Svanasana

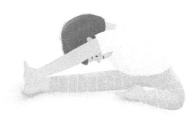

Dragonfly Pose: *Janu Sirsasana*

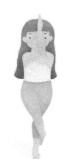

Eagle Pose: *Garudasana*

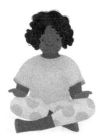

Flower Breath: *Sukhasana*

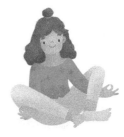

Flowering Lotus Pose: *Vikasitakamalasana*

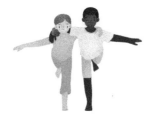

Flying Warriors Pose: *Virabhadrasana III*

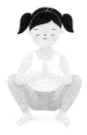

Frog Pose (Owl Pose): *Malasana*

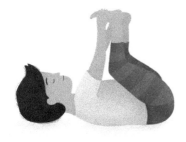

Happy Baby Pose: *Ananda Balasana*

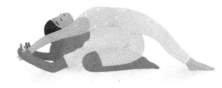

Lizard on a Rock (Fish Pose on Child's Pose): *Matsyasana* on *Balasana*

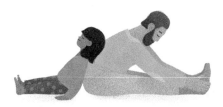

Lounge Chair (Fish Pose into Seated Forward Fold Pose): *Matsyasana* and *Paschimottanasana*

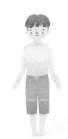

Mountain Pose: *Tadasana*

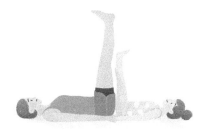

Partner Birthday Candle Pose (Partner Legs Up the Wall): *Viparita Karani*

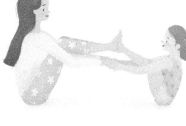

Partner Boat Pose: *Navasana*

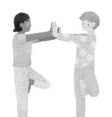

Partner Tree Pose: *Vrksasana*

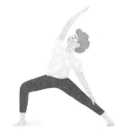

Peaceful Warrior Pose: *Shanti Virabhadrasana*

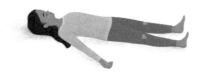

Relaxation Pose: *Savasana*

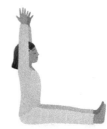

River Pose (Staff Pose): *Dandasana*

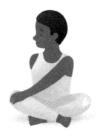

Seated Twist Pose:
Ardha Matsyendrasana

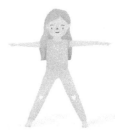

Standing Star Pose: *Utthita Tadasana*

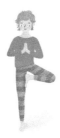

Tree Pose: *Vrksasana*

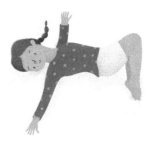

Twisty T Pose (Reclined Twist Pose):
Supta Matsyendrasana

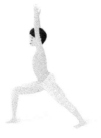

Warrior 1 Pose: *Virabhadrasana I*

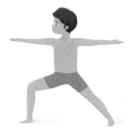

Warrior 2 Pose: *Virabhadrasana II*

Where to Learn More about Yoga

When I first started teaching yoga to kids more than 20 years ago, there were very few resources for kids. I lived in San Francisco where there was plenty of yoga, but not much for anyone who wasn't already fully grown. Now there are thousands of kids' yoga teachers around the world. There are YouTube channels (including mine!) as well as books, podcasts, and websites. There is no shortage of information to further your knowledge of bringing yoga to little ones. Here are some of my personal favorites. Once you start digging, you'll find what best suits you and your family's needs.

YouTube Channels

Cosmic Kids Yoga

If you have not done Cosmic Kids yet, you are in for a treat! This is a YouTube channel with hundreds of fun videos geared directly toward kids. Jamie will take you on interactive adventures to help kids build strength, balance, and confidence.
YouTube.com/c/cosmickidsyoga

Full of Joy Yoga

This is my YouTube channel. I offer a variety of five-minute mindfulness and yoga breaks to help kids get calm and focused and have fun. Make sure to check out all of my superhero breathing exercises!
YouTube.com/c/fullofjoyyoga

Kira Willey & Bari Koral

These are two of my favorite kids' yoga musicians. They have fun songs, meditations, and other resources especially for kids. Check out each of their YouTube channels for music that helps families find peace, calm, and fun. I even collaborated with Bari on her Super Me song: It is based on my superhero breaths!
YouTube.com/user/firefliesyoga
YouTube.com/user/barikoral
YouTube.com/watch?v=CDA8TbzOcms&list=PLh6hKQmd775iTmSj
Mw4saVBrGIW72zxTZ&index=1

Websites

Kids Yoga Stories

The ultimate resource for kids' yoga books, kids' yoga card decks, digital yoga cards, yoga posters and classroom yoga resources.
KidsYogaStories.com

Susan Verde

Susan's *I AM* series is a favorite along with her other magical stories. Her books support the work of teachers, librarians, and school mindfulness, yoga, and SEL programs.
SusanVerde.com/susans-books

Books

Calm Ninja: A Children's Book about Calming Your Anxiety Featuring the Calm Ninja Yoga Flow by Mary Nhin

Good Morning Yoga: A Pose-by-Pose Wake-Up Story by Mariam Gates

Good Night Yoga: A Pose-by-Pose Bedtime Story by Mariam Gates

A Little Calm Spot: A Story about Yoga and Feeling Focused by Diane Alber

Mindful Moves: Kid-Friendly Yoga and Peaceful Activities for a Happy, Healthy You by Nicole Cardoza

My Magic Breath: Finding Calm through Mindful Breathing by Nick Ortner and Alison Taylor

Our Family's Doing Yoga by SonJoria Sydnor

Yawning Yoga by Laurie Jordan

Yoga Friends: A Pose-by-Pose Partner Adventure for Kids by Mariam Gates and Rolf Gates

Acknowledgments

Thank you to all my teachers, mentors, friends, and collaborators in the kids' yoga biz. You have all made such an impact on my teaching, learning, and growing as I've embarked on my kids' yoga journey these last 20 years.

I have so much gratitude for all the parents who bring their kids to my classes, for the teachers and administrators who hire me and welcome me into their classrooms, and, finally, for the kiddos who bring me true joy daily with their creativity, curiosity, and endless love. You all make me feel like a rock star.

About the Author

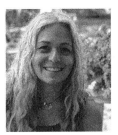

Lani Rosen-Gallagher, M.Ed., RCYT first incorporated yoga into her daily schedule while teaching first grade in Coney Island, New York. In 2004, Lani founded Full of Joy Yoga, a traveling yogi program, in San Francisco. Since 2006, she has organized and led her Full of Joy Yoga program and Mindful Yoga Breaks workshops all over the country. In 2007, she relocated to Connecticut, bringing her expertise to the East Coast. Her main goal is to get yoga and mindfulness into every school! Lani is always striving to improve the lives and futures of children, helping them laugh, love, and grow.

CPSIA information can be obtained
at www.ICGtesting.com
Printed in the USA
JSHW021655110722
27922JS00002B/7